Workout Meals

What and Why You Should Eat Before and After Your Exercise Routine to Burn Fat and Build Muscels Faster

Alicia Labert

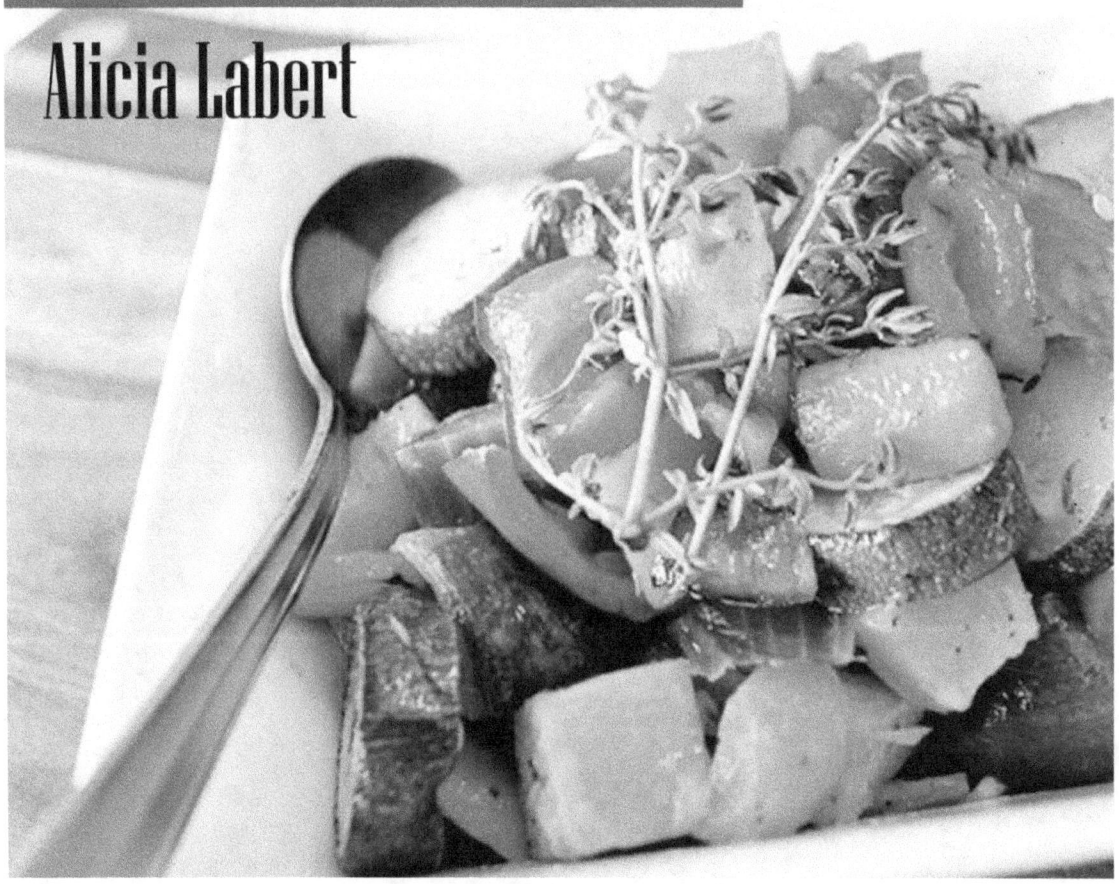

"The food you eat can either be safest and most powerful medicine or the slowest form of poison" – Ann Wigmore

Introduction

Every living creature has been eating food substance from the first day until the last day of its cycle. Humans are no exceptions; they need to eat food as well. But humans have developed exquisite taste that resulted in millions of food recipes. Yet it is disturbing that most of the people do not eat in healthy way. In result most people suffer from malnutrition, underweight or obesity.

When healthy food is consumed in the right quantities, it isn't very difficult to lead a healthy lifestyle by developing a body that is fit. Not many people know how to do it. This book explains the role of food in your life and its importance in attaining the body you want. Since each person has a unique body as well as taste, eating habits with appropriate food substances of your liking should be included in your diet.

It is very easy to sit on a couch and eat all the junk you find and subsequently gain a very unhealthy body but it takes a lot of determination and grit to take your body in the opposite direction and make it healthy. Once you get the hang of it, you will actually enjoy the process of consuming healthy foods and you may even start experimenting with various food substances in the process of making new recipes. Always remember the fact that a healthy body leads to a healthy lifestyle, and a healthy lifestyle leads to prosperity and happiness.

This book is intended to bring awareness among the readers about the role of food in the process of transforming the body. If you want to reduce your weight, fat burning food are available, if you want to become more muscular, good exercise and eating right will do it. Whatever your goal might be, eating the right food will change your life.

Eat according to the workout.

Consume the wrong food before your workout and you will feel lethargic and won't be able to perform the workout to your full extent; eat the wrong food after you exercise and all the effort put into the workout will never yield any significant result. There seems to be a million ways to fail while only a handful will get you the results.

Food substances are consumed by humans with a goal of digesting it and producing energy to perform their day to day activities. But when the wrong food substance is consumed in wrong quantities, your body will slowly degrade over time causing irreparable damage to itself. But for people with a goal to take control of their body, eating right is the first step in attaining the body they want.

There are a lot of health supplements that target the body before and after a workout, they produce results as long as your take these health supplements, but the day you stop taking them is the day your body will start to lose its fitness and shape. That is why I encourage all the readers to build their body using natural food substances. Also I can never stress enough on the fact that the sleep cycle of 8 hours and right food intake is as essential as the workout itself. These three consist of the process of muscle growth.

Pre workout foods for strength training workout.

A great man said, "Abs are built in the kitchen as much as they are in the gym". I have seen many people who work out on empty stomach and complain that the results are not what they expect. That is why you should never workout on empty stomach.

But what is the role of the food consumed before an actual workout?

The main purpose of the food before you exercise is to help you to perform the workout efficiently. It will help you to prepare for the incoming muscle stress during a workout; it regulates the blood flow and makes loads of energy available for working out while still being light on the stomach and your body. You can lift heavier weights in a better way with pre workouts.

Having pre workout meal before exercise actually increases your cardio vascular activity. It fuels your body to perform the upcoming workout to your full extent. But there is a time limit for it, pre workout meals should be consumed 30 to 60 mins before the workout to stay optimized.

There are tons of recipes for the pre workout meals and some of them don't need much time to prepare:

1. Bananas or any fruit will do
2. Whole wheat bread
3. Power bars
4. Milk
5. Raw egg
6. Nuts
7. Yams
8. Peanut butter with brown bread

If you have time to prepare a recipe, there are lots available, here are some of them:

Banana smoothie

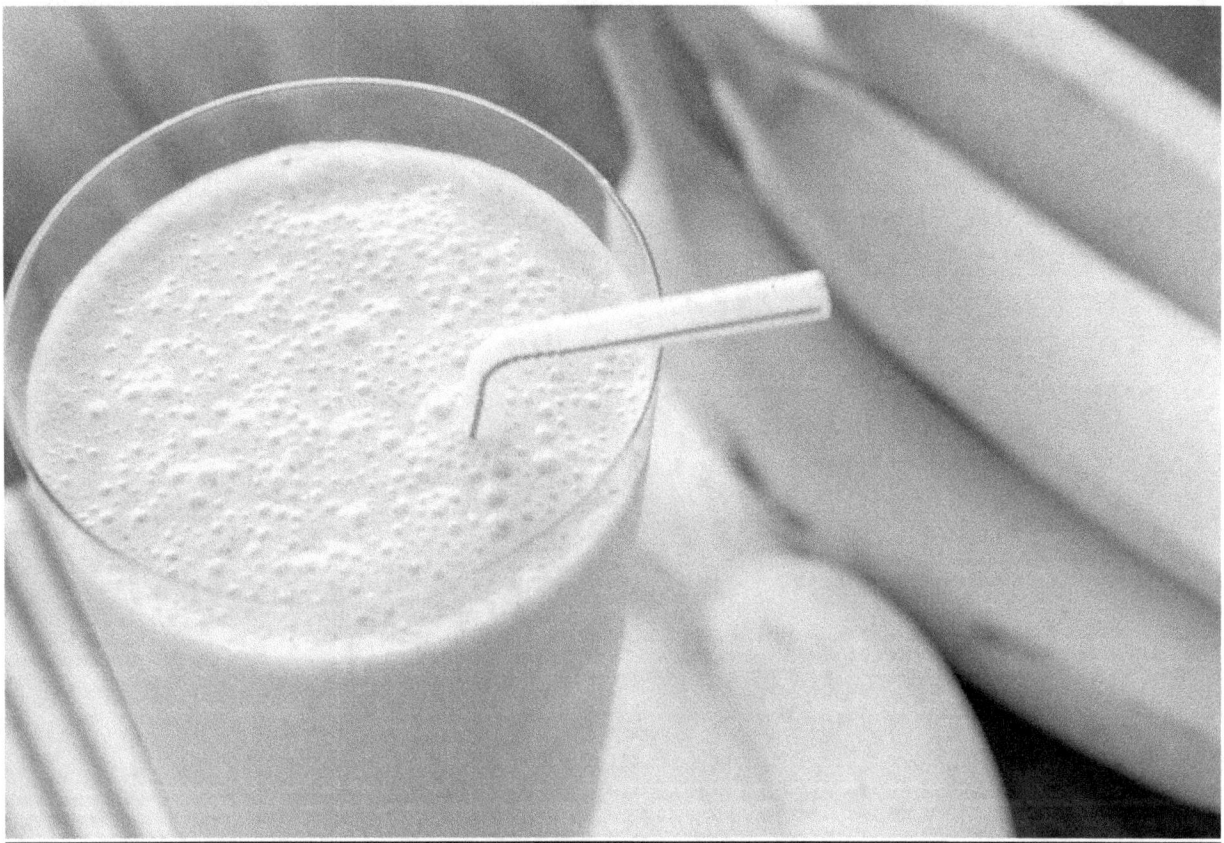

Ingredients

- banana
- fat free milk
- cocoa powder
- chocolate syrup
- mint extract
- unsaturated sugar
- ice cubes
- sweetened cream

Preparation method

1. Take a large banana and cut it into pieces, sprinkle it with powdered sugar and cocoa power.
2. Put it in the freezer for about 3 hours until it is rock solid.

3. Take this rock solid banana pieces and put it into a blender along with ice cubes, mint extract, cocoa power, chocolate power and milk, blend all the ingredients until it becomes semi liquid. Pour it in a glass.
4. Drink when chilled.

Oat meal

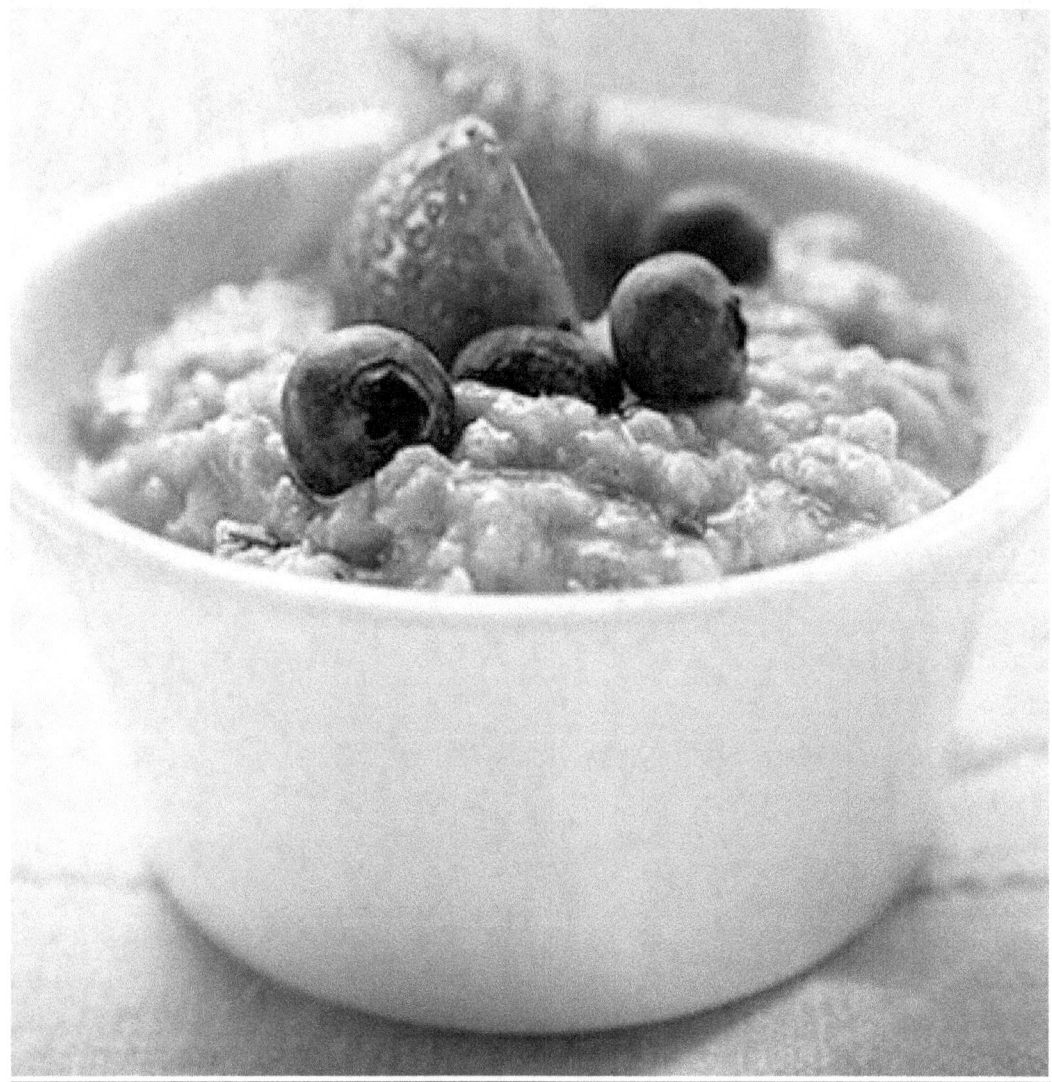

Ingredients

- Quaker oats
- Water
- Almonds
- Walnuts

- Cashew nuts
- Sugar

<u>Preparation method</u>

1. Place a pan on the heater, pour 200 ml of water and bring it to boil.
2. Add 2 teaspoon of sugar and Quaker oats.
3. You can add salt combined with other spices instead of sugar to give the recipe an entire different twist.
4. Wait 2 mins and place the lid for about 5 mins.
5. After that, remove the lid and put in the nuts. You can add blueberries and it will still taste good for the sugar oats recipe.
6. Put out the fire and place the lid for about 2 mins before consuming with fresh fruit juice.

Egg toast

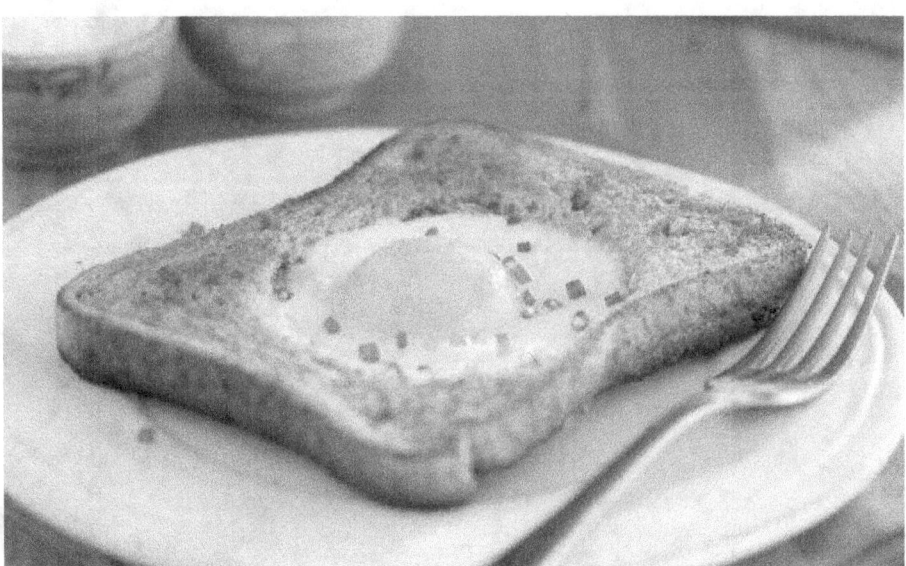

<u>Ingredients</u>

- Egg
- Salt
- brown bread toast
- Parsley

<u>Preparation method</u>

1. Prepare a brown bread, or whole wheat bread or multi grain bread toast of 3 slices.
2. Heat a pan; spray the olive oil lightly so that the egg doesn't stick to the pan.
3. Break the egg in the pan and sprinkle a pinch of salt on it.
4. Do not disturb or turn the egg.
5. After 2 mins, place the egg on the toast.
6. Sprinkle parsley on it.
7. Eat while it is still hot.

Berry blast

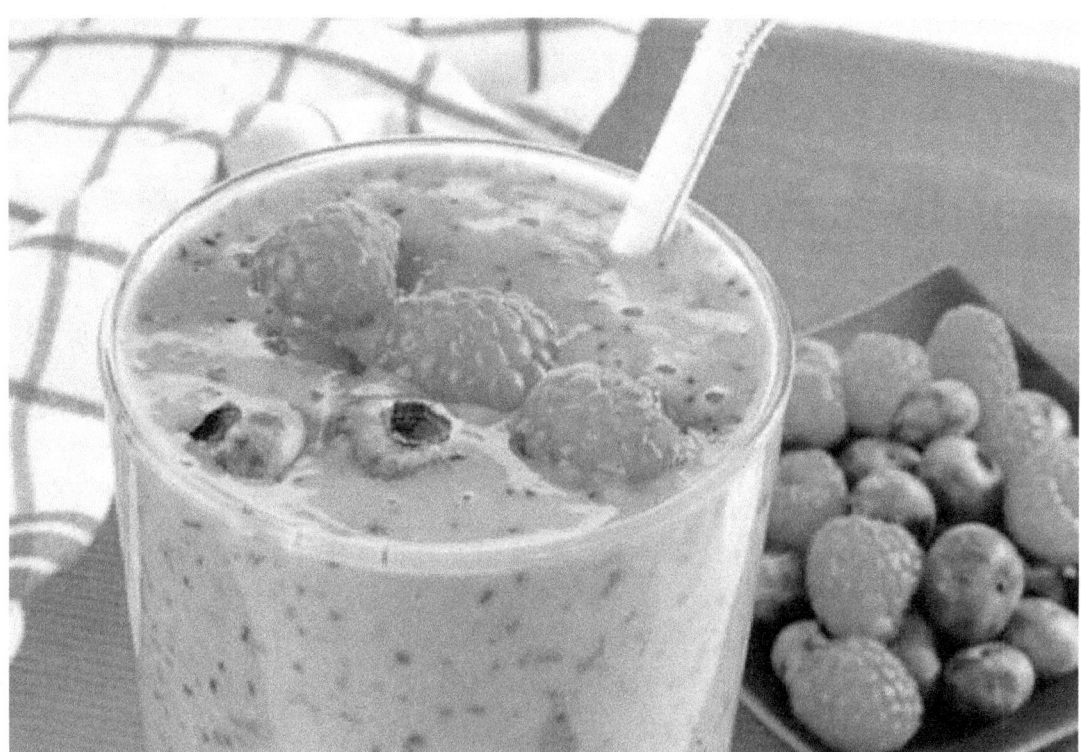

<u>Ingredients</u>

- Skimmed milk
- Berries of your choice
- Ice cubes
- Cardamom
- Mint leaves
- Sugar

Preparation method

1. Take a blender and put in some ice cubes.
2. Pour the skimmed milk and put berries into the blender.
3. At last, add the sugar and cardamom.
4. Blend it until the ice cubes are crushed properly and the berries are invisible.
5. Pour it into the glass and top it with mint leaves for added flavor.

Post workout foods for strength training workout

While the pre workout meals are aimed at providing maximum energy to the body while working out without being heavy on the stomach, the post workouts repair the body that has been damaged while exercising. The science behind working out is that when you perform strength training exercises, the muscles will be subjected to continuous voluntary stress that causes small tears in it.
These tears are what causes the muscular mass to grow in size. They happen when the tears are repaired by protein that has been accumulated by digesting the food consumed. Simply speaking

More tears = more muscle repair = more muscular growth

The science behind efficient muscle building techniques is that when you have 1 or 2 big meals that have lots of protein, carbs and good fat in it, your body will only utilize a part of it and the rest goes down the drain. Instead, it is best to have 5 to 6 small meals in the day.

The reason is that when you have a big meal, the body takes up what is necessary for the time period and rejects the rest. But after some time it will need the essential nutrients and proteins again. But this time, those are not available and the muscle repairing stops, resulting in degradation of the body. When you take meals 5 to 6 times a day, it will provide small amount of nutrients that the body utilizes and nutrients are not wasted. After some time when the body needs the nutrients again, you will have another meal and provide the nutrients thus continuing the process of muscle repairing and growing.

As far as dieting is concerned, it isn't simply eating some super foods that helps the body but growing the body while simultaneously removing the toxic waste. Fruits and juicing will help you to detox the body while still providing the essentials for muscle growth. In some cases, fasting for one day a week also helps tremendously to detox. Understand the needs of your body to mold it in a way you want it to be.

The following are the recipes that will help you to repair your muscles after a workout with right amount of sleep.

Pepper egg burrito

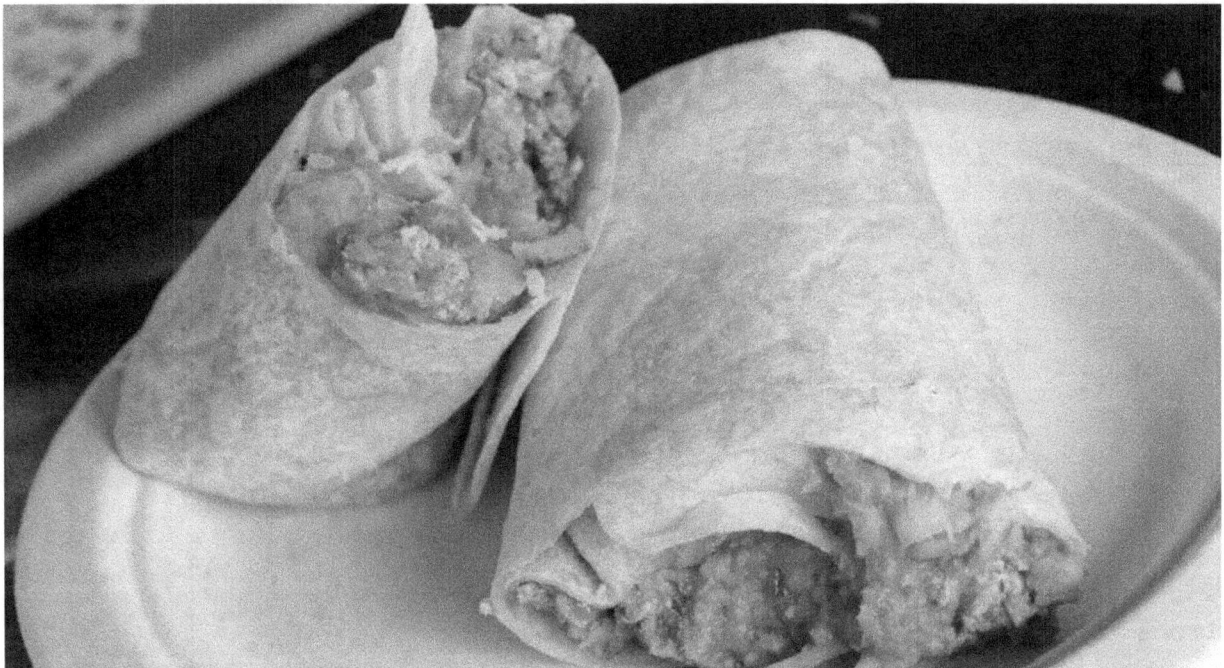

Ingredients

- Whole grain bread wrapped into sandwich half
- Eggs without yolk
- Eggs with yolk
- Finely chopped onions
- Green, red and yellow peppers
- Fat free cheese in shredded form
- jalapeno pepper cut into small pieces
- Black beans
- Salsa which is spiced and canned

Preparation method

1. Put in the sandwich wraps into a toaster which is covered with heat wraps and let it toast nice for a full 4 minutes.
2. Whisk the combination of 4 eggs without yolk, 2 eggs with yolk, beans and cheese into a smooth mixture.
3. Put in small quantity of olive oil into a non-stick frying pan and let it heat for a minute; when heated, put in the egg and bean mixture and let it cook for a full 2 minute.
4. Put in the peppers which, chopped into fine pieces on top of omelet and let it cook until it is done.

5. Spread the spicy salsa on top of the sandwich slice wraps, divide the omelet into the number of pieces you want and spread on top of the wraps. Have it while hot or wrap it into heat wraps if you want to have it later.

Smoked chicken salad

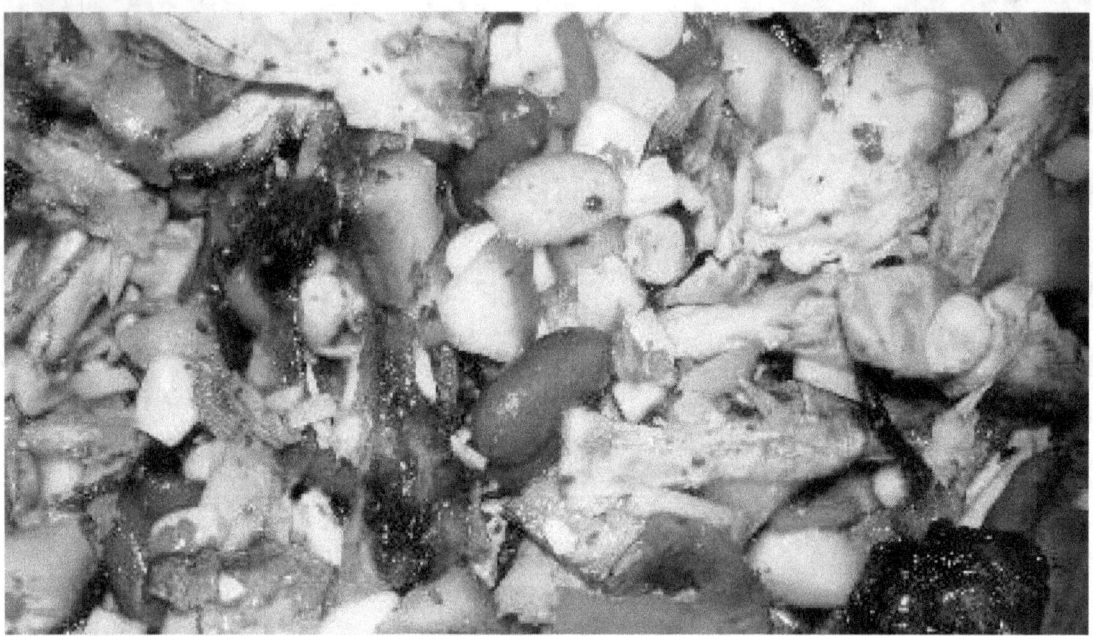

Ingredients

- 10 ml adobo sauce
- Full chicken
- Roasted nuts of your choice
- Water
- Boiled potatoes
- parsley
- Chopped herbs
- Soy sauce
- Washed and salted lentils

Preparation method

1. Coat the full chicken lightly with olive oil and put in some herbs and onions in the middle and barbeque it until it is nicely cooked with the entire flavor, then cut them into pieces of sizes of your desire.
2. Take a pressure cooker and put in the lentils, adobo sauce and various herbs; herbs are good for health, so take whatever you like in whatever quantity you want and cook them until they are nicely done.

3. If you don't have a pressure cooker, take a cooking bowl and put lentils, herbs and adobo sauce i and cook for 10 minutes until the water is evaporated and the lentils are thoroughly cooked.
4. After that, add the boiled potatoes and let the lentils be in the steam for a few minutes.
5. Transfer the chicken into a plate and mix it well with the roasted nuts and parsley.
6. Mix the soy sauce into the chicken well for the tangy flavor.
7. Place the chicken on the lentils and have them hot.

Mushroom ham sandwich

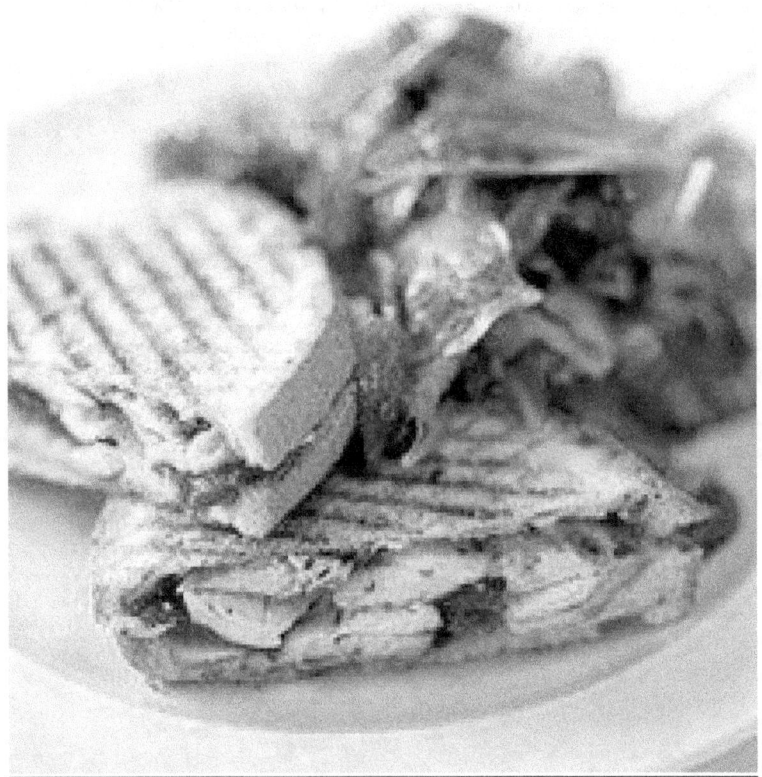

Ingredients

- Mushrooms
- Oil spray
- Onions
- Ham
- Grain bread
- Greek yogurt
- Chicken
- Pepper cheese

<u>Preparation method</u>

1. Take the mushrooms and wash them thoroughly in salt water, boil them for 10 minute until they are soft. Drain the water and let them cool in a bowl.
2. Heat a non-stick pan and spray some of the oil spray. Put in sliced ham and chicken, mixing them thoroughly and after a few minutes add the oil and Greek yogurt.
3. By now the mushroom must have cooled down, place the bread slices onto an aluminum wraps, spread the pepper cheese on them, you can take mayo if you prefer it.
4. Cut the mushroom into fine pieces and place them on the slices, put in adequate quantity of the chicken ham mixture.
5. Garnish them with raw onion and parsley before placing the top slice of sandwich and sealing them in the aluminum wrap.

Papaya-strawberry shake

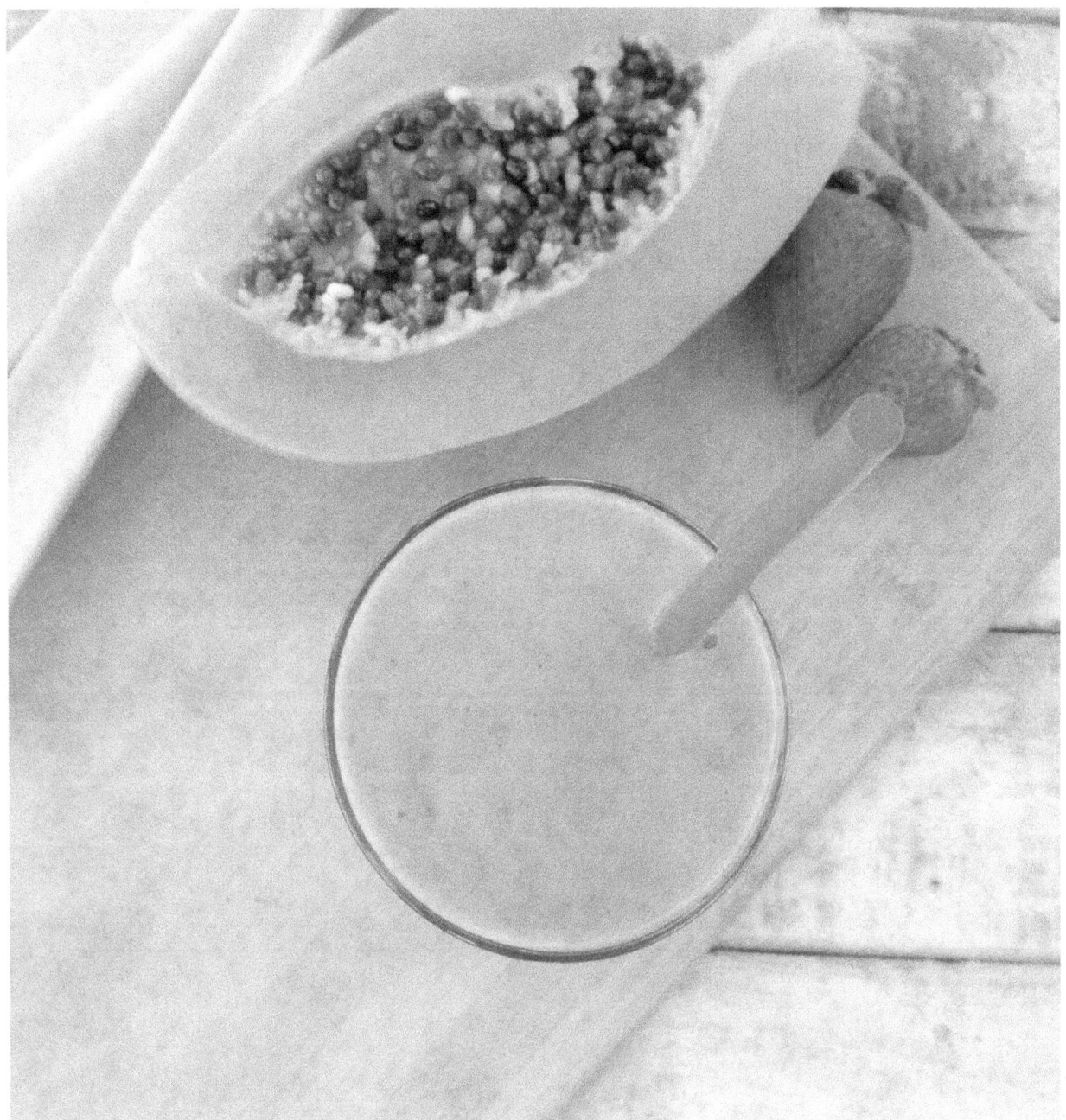

<u>Ingredients</u>

- Few strawberries
- Papaya
- Greek yogurt (fat free or low fat)
- Ice

<u>Preparation method</u>

1. Remove the stem from the strawberries and the skin from the papaya.
2. Cut them into small pieces.
3. Put everything into the blender including yogurt and ice.
4. Blend until a smooth shake is formed.
5. Have it when chilled.

<u>Salmon fillets with maple flavor</u>

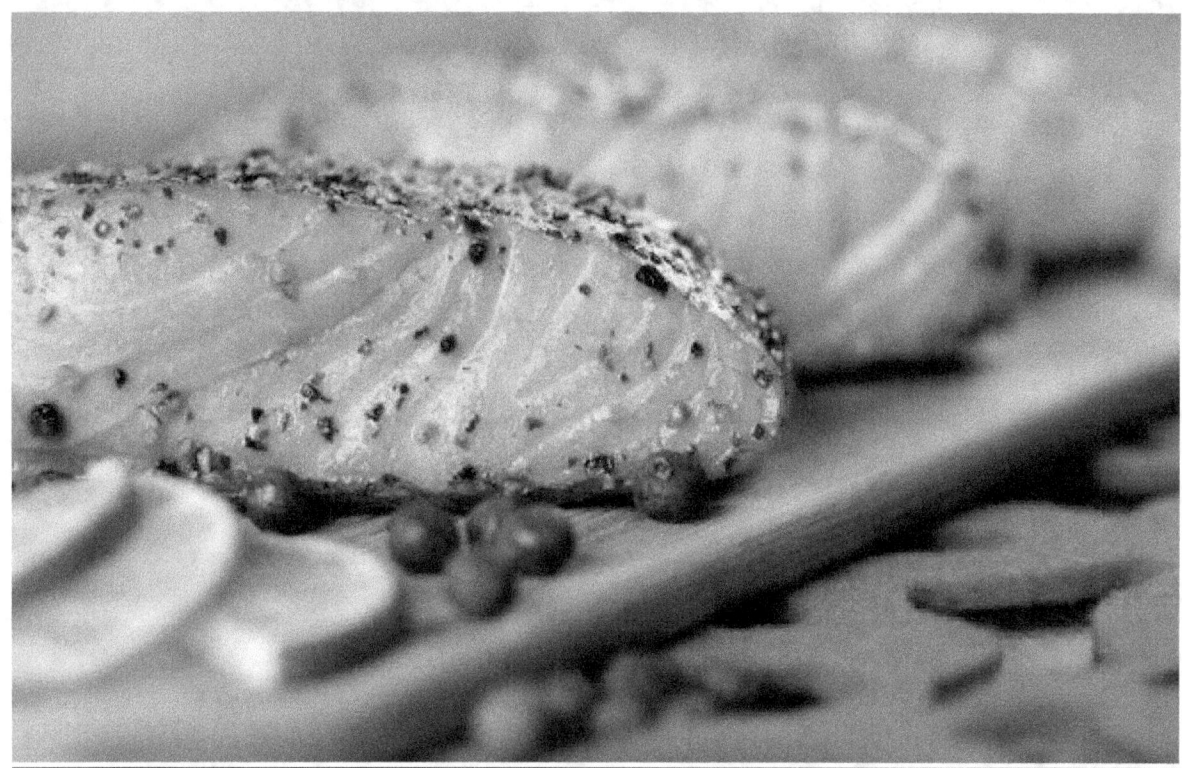

<u>Ingredients</u>

- Vinegar
- Oil spray
- Pepper to taste
- Salmon-fillets
- Soy sauce
- Herbs of your liking
- Peppers of various types
- Nuts especially cashew
- Maple syrup

<u>Preparation method</u>

1. In a pan, put in the soy sauce, vinegar, a little bit of oil, salt and pepper and let it heat until a thick mixture is formed.
2. Now take a non-stick pan and lightly coat it with oil spray and place the salmon-fillet onto the pan. Turn it over after exactly 30 seconds on medium flame.
3. Now the light crispy top will be coated with the maple mixture which we have prepared earlier. Immediately turn it over and again coat the light crisp underside with the same mixture.
4. We will turn off the heat. Let the salmon be on the pan for a minute. It to fully cook in the inside.
5. Take a large container, put in two table spoons of maple syrup, a few roasted nuts and cooked peppers. I personally mixed them with mint leaves as they bring extra flavor to the dish.
6. Mix them well to form a thick paste which has to be evenly spread onto the base of the container, place the fillets on top of them and serve.

Homemade protein bar

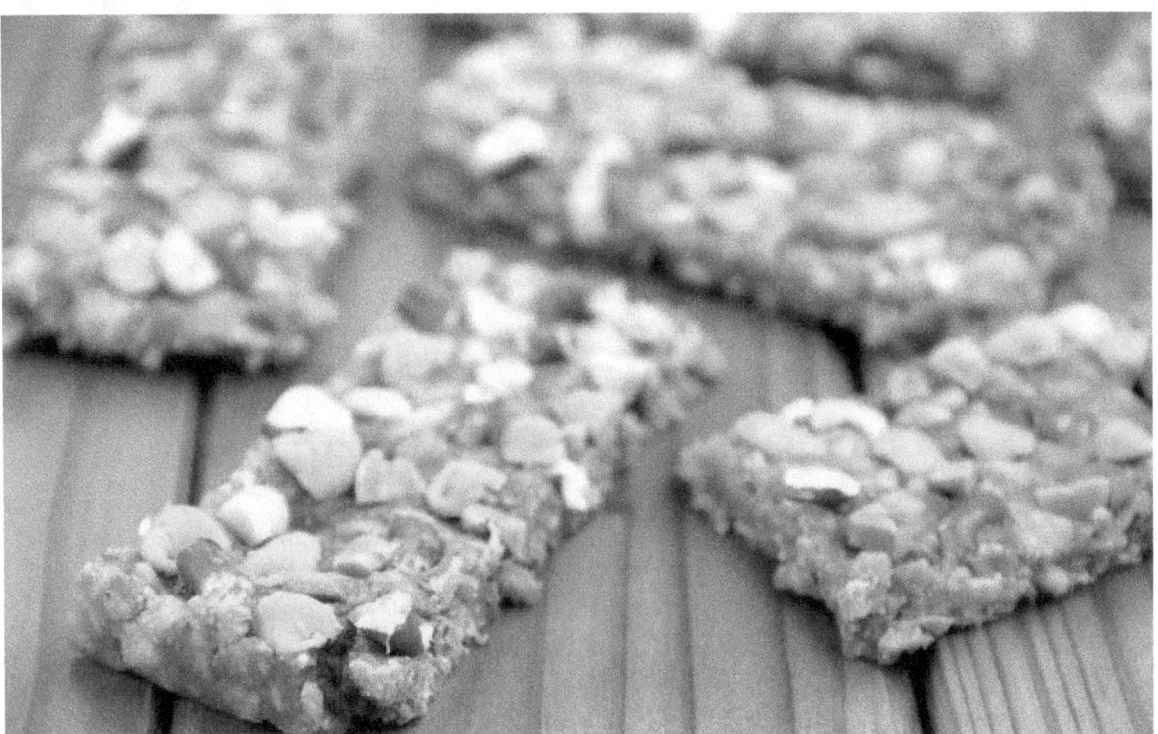

<u>Ingredients</u>

- Peanut butter
- Peanuts
- Soy crisps
- Protein powder
- Pretzel twists

Preparation method

1. Take a baking pan and grease it lightly with oil spray.
2. Put the soy crisps into the blender and blend them roughly so that bit remains.
3. Put the content into a bowl and add the protein powder into the mixture. Mix them well.
4. Add the peanut butter and some water so as to make a semi liquid mixture. Cook it on medium flame for 5 minutes.
5. Transfer the content of the cooking pot into the baking pan. Sprinkle loads of peanuts, pretzel twists and almonds which are roughly beaten. Now let it cool for about 30 minutes before cutting it into small pieces and consuming them. Adding honey will not only increase the bar's sweetness but also health benefits.

Whole wheat linguine with shrimp

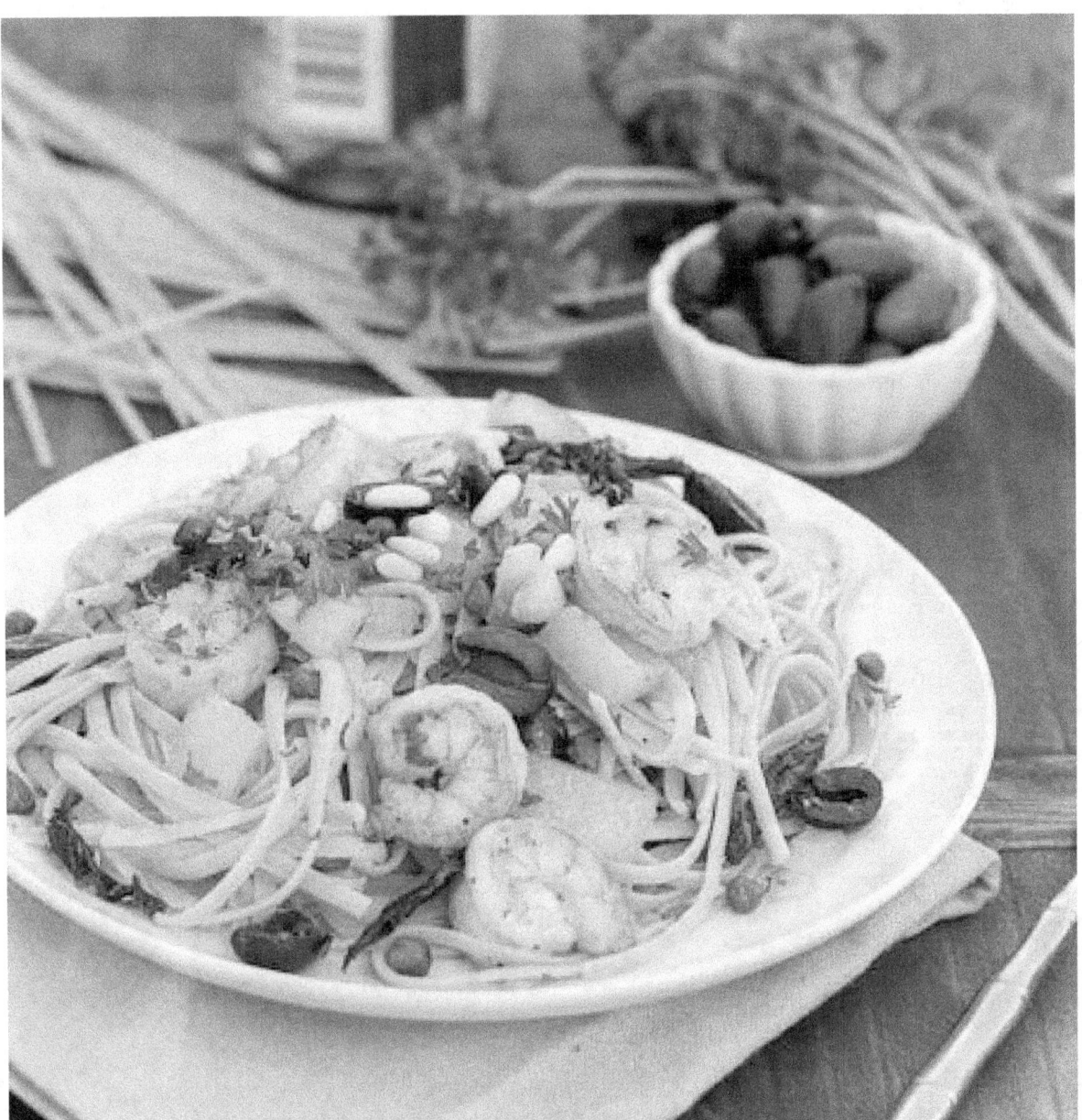

Ingredients

- 10 oz. of whole wheat linguine
- Shrimp (any other sea food if you prefer)
- Olive oil
- Onion
- Ginger
- Garlic
- Salt and pepper
- Fresher peppers

- Chili flakes
- Roasted almonds
- Parsley

Preparation method

1. Peel shrimps and cook them in a pressure cooker.
2. Heat 2 table spoons of olive oil in a nonstick pan and season the shrimp when they become cold. Add salt and pepper. Cook on medium flame for 3 minutes until they are almost ready. Be careful not to burn shrimps.
3. Put the contents aside and add a table spoon of olive oil, onion, finely chopped ginger and garlic, peppers in the same pan. Sauté for few minutes before adding the linguine along with chilli flakes. Cook for 5 minutes on low flame.
4. Now mix shrimps and linguine along with roasted almonds and parsley in a bowl with a spoon. Set aside for 2 minutes before consuming.

How to burn fat and get into the fittest shape of your life?

You eat food and food has calories. Every physical labor you do requires calories. These calories are the unit of energy contained in your body. When some of them are left over without being used, they will be stored and converted into fat cells by the body with a purpose that it can be used when the energy intake is scarce.

Fat is important for the body's normal functioning and survival. The purpose of the good fat is to produce energy and enable other organs to do their jobs when the energy levels are depleted. We cannot live without good fats but we need it only in small quantities. All the accumulated fat on your waist is not necessary for your survival.

Our bodies require small amounts of good fat to function properly and help the body to resist diseases. But the food we eat sometimes is to be blamed for the imbalance due to its content of saturated fat and unwanted substances which can be harmful.

Understanding how the fat is burnt

The fat burning process can be explained in a single sentence. "**Consume fewer calories than what you need and the body will automatically burn fat for you**".

All physical work requires energy and you provide that energy by consuming food. When you eat more calories than what is required, that energy is converted to fat. We will reverse the process so that the same body which is making fat will actually destroy it. Here's how your body will do it with process reversal method. You will perform your regular tasks as before and your body will spend its usual amount of calories but this time you will perform cardio exercises for a small amount of time which requires energy. To do this, your body will convert the stored fat into energy by a reverse chemical reaction and use the energy to perform the task.

The process will be slow..... Dead slow. Do not get cheated by the television advertising promising to reduce a pound in a day. Quick reduction of belly fat is a myth and it cannot be done without surgical procedures. It all takes work and sweat, but the result is worth it.

When you spend more calories than what you eat, your body compensates the energy difference by burning fat and producing energy from it. Now fat is stored not only in your belly but is spread all over your body. So when fat is burned, it is first burned in all the places except your belly. When all fat in your body has been burned, your body finally utilizes the belly fat. This is the reason why many people give up because of low results after weeks and weeks of workout. It is painstaking to not reduce the belly fat even after weeks of workout but once you burn fat all over it will eventually start burning fat you're your stomach. Patience and perseverance is what you should keep in mind if you want to have the dream body which you desire.

So how is that certain type of foods help you burn fat while other makes you fat?

Some foods, when consumed regularly with combination of other food will actually increase your metabolism rate to such an extent that they will slowly burn your fat. Fat burning food method is nothing but the process where the energy required to digest that food particles is more than energy given by digesting them.

Foods which are very hard to digest require high energy to break them down, but give out low energy after digestion. These are called **fat reduction or fat burning food.**

Fat burning foods

Here is the list of foods which can help you reduce fat:

- Ginger
- Fat free milk
- Olive oil
- Citrus fruits like lemon and oranges
- Green tea
- Egg whites
- Salmon, tuna and mackerel
- Garlic
- Oatmeal
- Whole grain such as brown rice, quinoa and whole grain cereal
- Almonds and other nuts
- Apples
- Grape fruit
- Chicken and turkey breast
- Pears
- Mushrooms
- Lentils
- Hot peppers
- Broccoli
- Spinach and other veggies
- Avocado
- Greek yogurt
- Blueberries and other berries
- Peanut butter
- Legumes
- Soy protein
- Cinnamon

Recipes to help you burn fat

Broccoli egg toast (post workout)

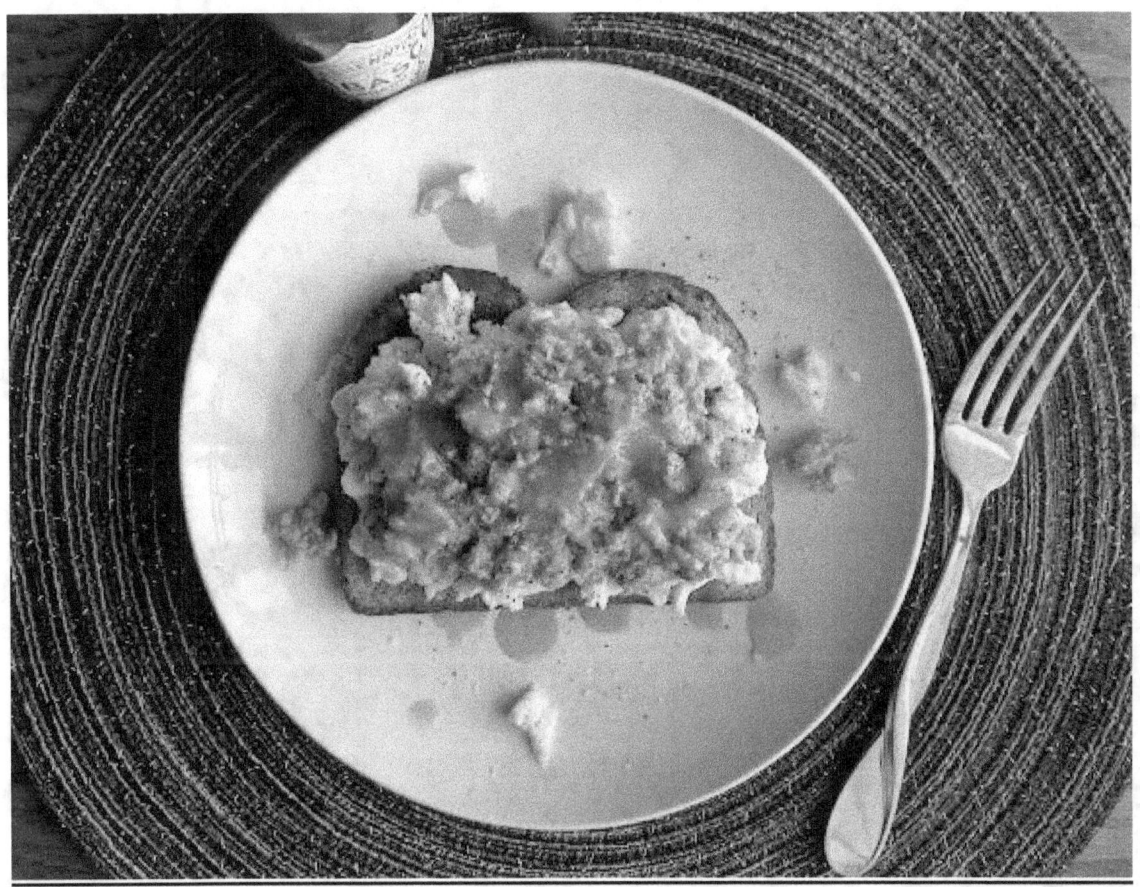

Ingredients

- Olive oil
- Toasted whole grain bread slices
- Low fat cheese
- Beaten eggs as much as you like
- Sliced broccoli
- Powdered dill

<u>Preparation method</u>

1. Heat the pan then spray it lightly with olive oil. Add chopped broccoli and leave until properly cooked.
2. Beat the eggs and add the cheese. Put in few spices if you desire. Add this mixture with the broccoli and let it simmer until cooked.
3. Have it with the toasted bread slices while hot.

Green tea drink (pre workout)

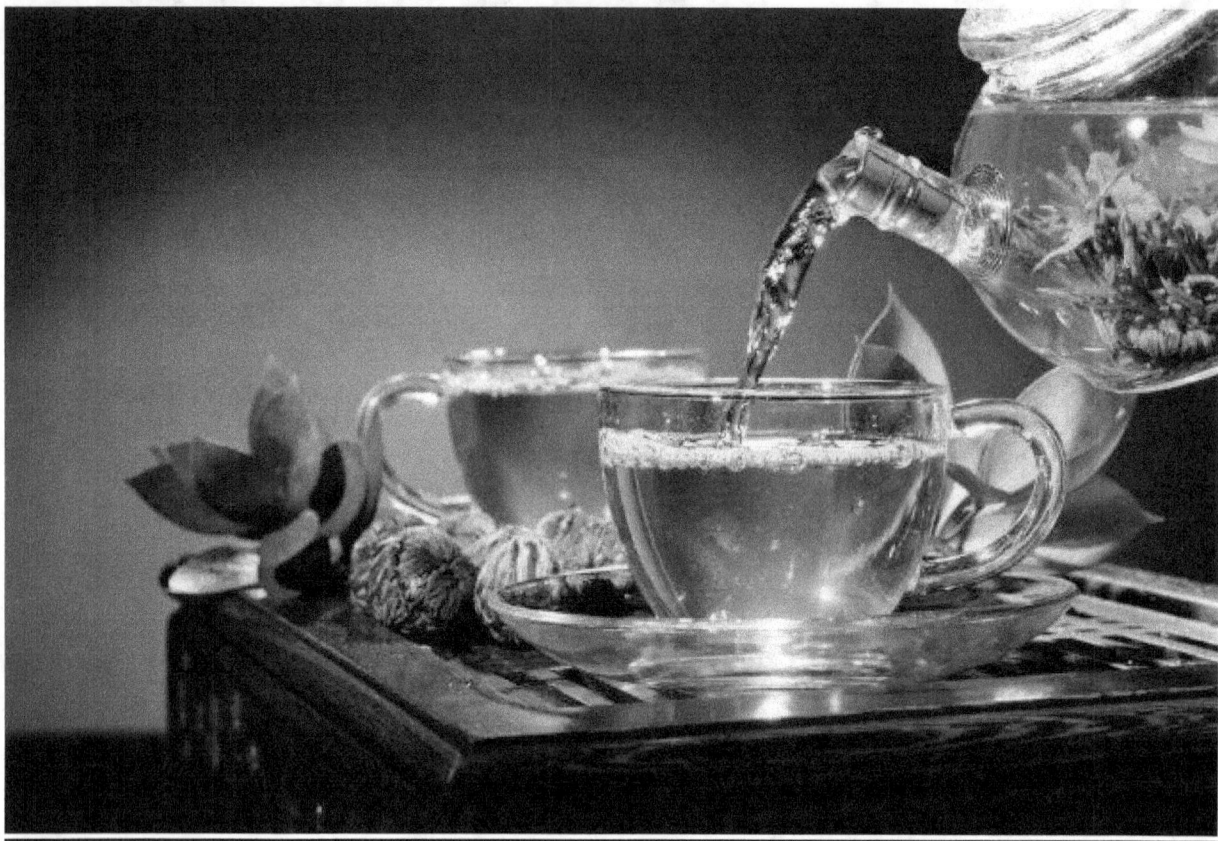

<u>Ingredients</u>

- Water
- Green tea
- A little pepper
- Lemon
- Honey as much as you like
- Sliced pear, one in number
- Greek yogurt
- Plenty of ice cubes

<u>Preparation method</u>

1. Boil the water and put in the green tea along with honey. Let it get slightly warm. Careful not to boil it entirely.
2. Let it cool for a few minutes. When the tea reaches room temperature, add all the mentioned ingredients and blend it nicely.
3. Have it cold.

Berry toast (post workout)

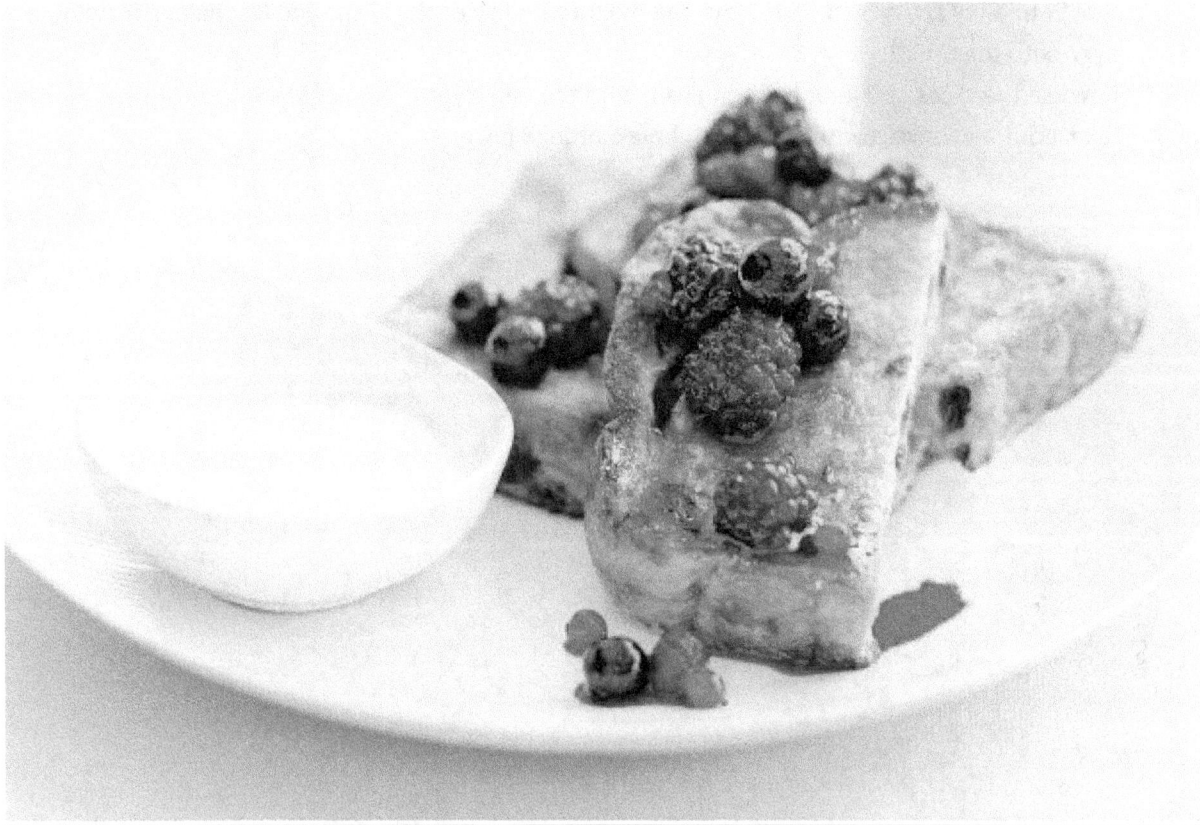

<u>Ingredients</u>

- Any berry you like, blueberry in this case
- Low fat cheese
- Milk which is fat free
- Little sugar
- Two eggs without yolk
- Egg with yolk

- Any berry essence
- Olive oil
- Bread made of whole wheat

Preparation method

1. Make a nice and smooth mixture by blending berries with 200 ml of milk, cheese and sugar. Taste it and put the sugar until it is sweet.
2. Add whole eggs, eggs without yolk and 250ml of milk in a blender to make a smooth mixture.
3. Spread berry mixture on top of the bread.
4. Heat a nonstick frying pan. Spread the olive oil lightly and place the bread slices onto them. Keep it till they are brown. Put in the egg mixture on top of the slices and let the egg form a layer onto the bread.
5. Reverse the slices and let it happen again with the egg layer.
6. Take it out and have it with freshly squeezed orange juice.

Shakshuka (post workout)

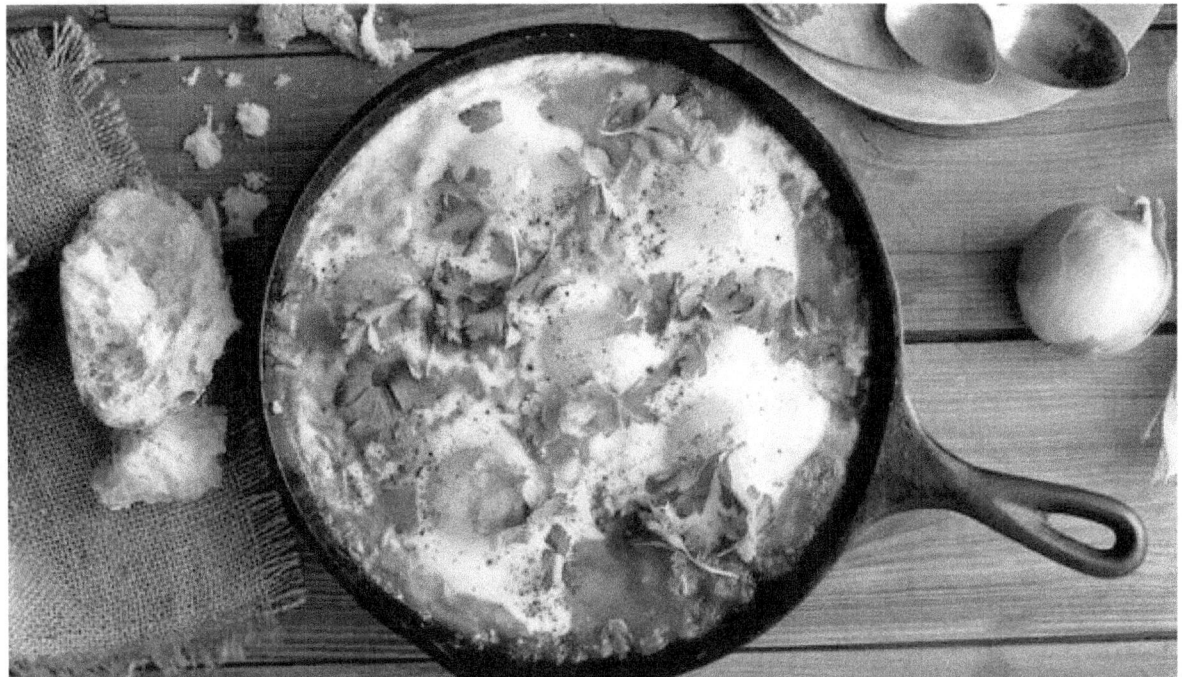

Ingredients

- Oil spray
- Rock salt to taste
- Tomato puree and also fresh tomatoes
- peppers
- Ginger and garlic which are finely chopped
- Cumin seeds
- red onions
- Jalapenos
- Half a dozen full eggs
- parsley
- Mozzarella cheese

Preparation method

1. This dish has few layers
2. First layer: heat a cooking pot with light oil in it. Put in the medium sized pepper pieces with onions and a pinch of salt.
3. Leave them until onions turn to golden brown. Be careful to not burn peppers.

4. Second, add the finely chopped ginger and garlic pieces. Mix the content well so that the flavor is evenly distributed.

5. Third, squeeze the fresh tomatoes in a bowl. Put in the tomato puree into the cooking pot while slowly mixing the contents. After 2 minutes on medium flame, just put in the squeezed tomatoes along with the extracts and boil it for about 4 minutes.

6. The final step is to add eggs. This is the distinguishing feature of shakshuka. Just crack the eggs on top of the mixture in the cooking pot without disturbing the yellow yolk; lightly spread the egg white with a spoon so that they form a thin layer on top of the tomato mixture.

7. Cover the lid and leave it for about 10 minutes on low flame which will enable the eggs to cook slowly and nicely on the top, but be careful not to cook the eggs fully. They must stay half cooked in the center of the yolk.

8. Have it as it is or with a slice of bread.

Pita chips with hummus (post workout)

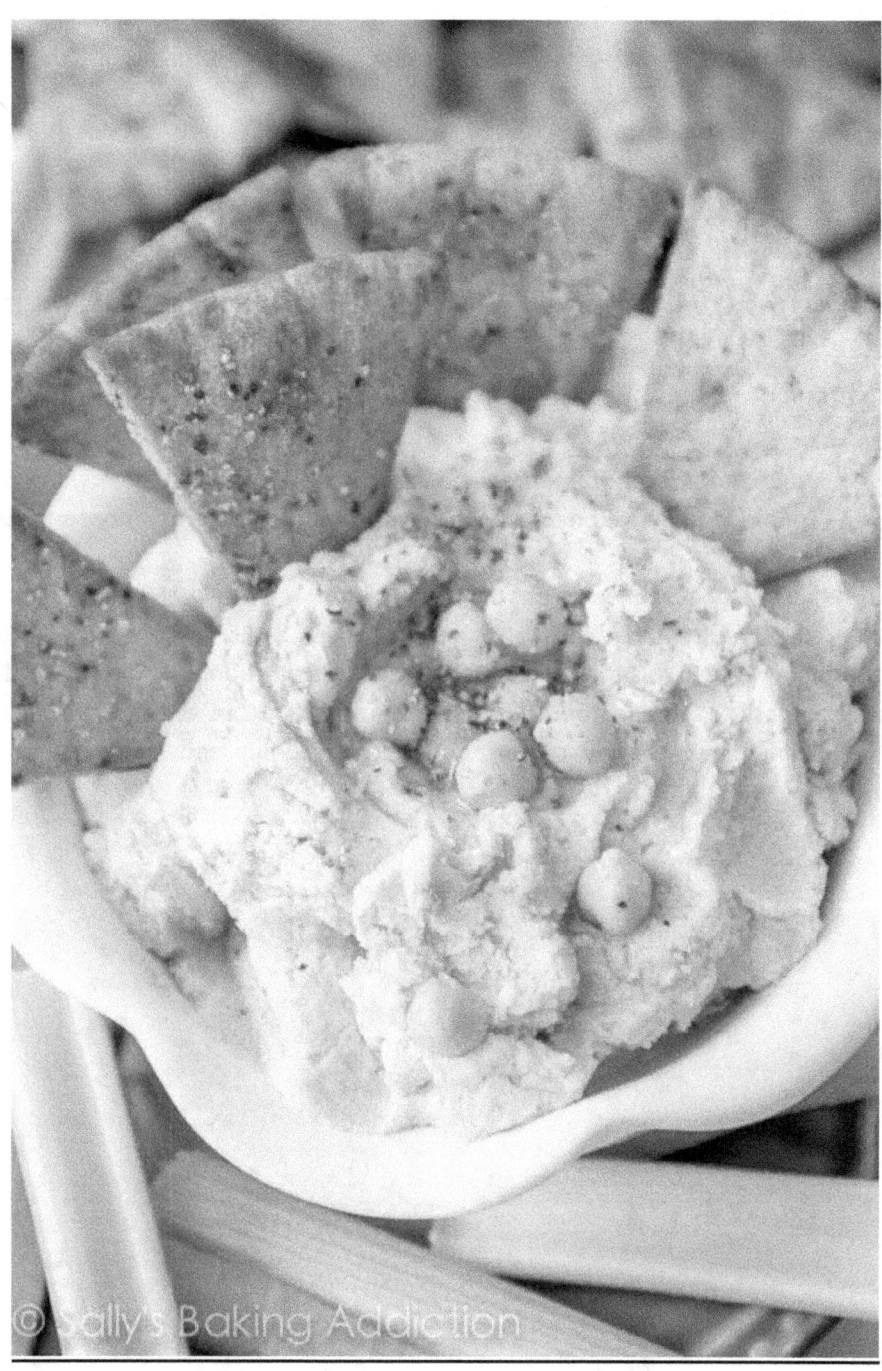

<u>Ingredients</u>

<u>For pita chips</u>

- Pitas
- Olive oil

- Finely chopped garlic
- Salt and pepper

For hummus

- Boiled and drained chickpeas
- Chopped garlic
- Freshly squeezed lemon juice
- Half a cup tahini
- Parsley and cumin seeds

Preparation method

1. Pre heat the oven to 350 degrees Fahrenheit.
2. Cut pitas into triangular shape.
3. Mix olive oil, salt, pepper, chopped or pasted garlic, and pita triangles. Mix them well and place them in the baking sheet in to the oven. Leave them for 15 minutes before removing. These are the pita chips.
4. While the chips are being baked, prepare hummus.
5. In a food processor, put in the boiled chickpeas, peppers, garlic. Make a thick paste.
6. Then add some water to this thick paste, tahini, and 2 table spoons of olive oil and lemon juice. Mix it well so that the thick paste turns to smooth mixture. Transfer it to a bowl. Taste it and add salt and lemon juice as per you liking. Sprinkle with cumin seeds and parsley.
7. Serve pita chips with hummus.

Flavored tacos (post workout)

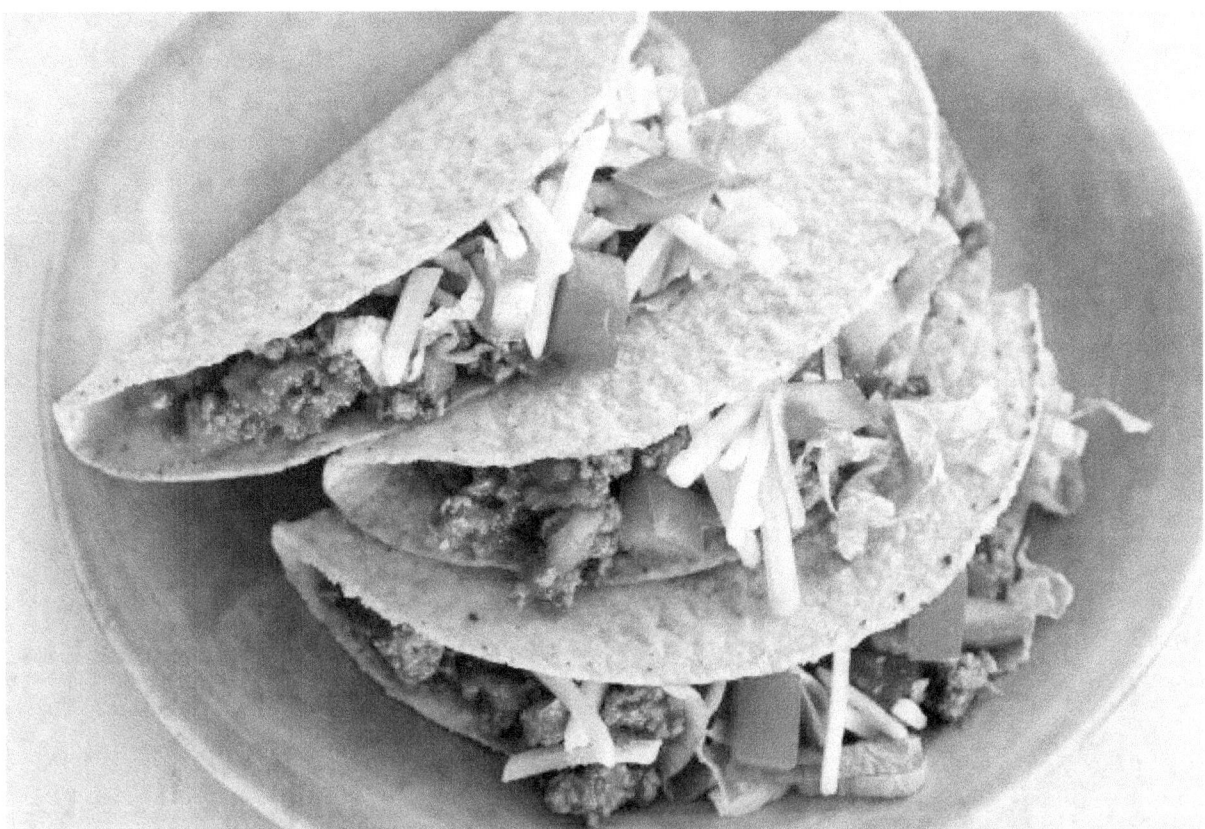

Ingredients

- Oil spray
- Low fat cream
- Adobo sauce
- Chile
- Tacos
- Ginger
- Garlic
- Onions
- Salt
- Pepper
- Lentils
- Tomato
- cheese
- Lettuce
- Broth of your wish
- Cheddar

Preparation method

1. Heat a large cooking pot with small amount of oil in it.
2. Put in finely chopped ginger and garlic along with slices of onion. Cook this mixture until the onions turn into golden brown.
3. Mix the tacos along with lentils. Allow it to cook until the lentils are almost cooked. When this is done, mix the broth of your taste into the tacos and allow them to simmer.
4. Mix the low fat cream with a little bit of pepper and adobo sauce in a container.
5. After the lentils are cooked, mix them with broth.
6. When the flavor smells good, add previously prepared cream mixture on the top. Cut the tomatoes and place them on the top and close the lid to cook the entire mixture for about 2 minutes on medium flame before consumption.

Multi fruit frappe (post workout)

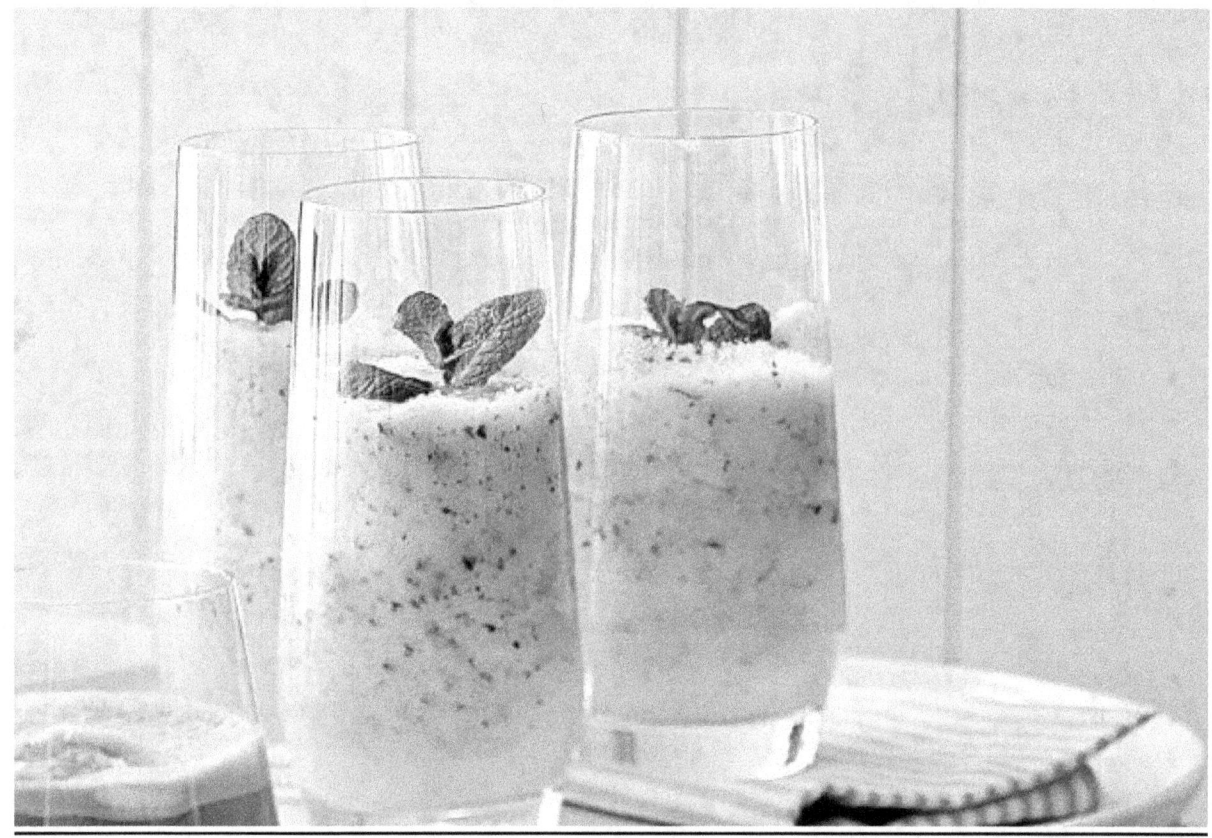

Ingredients

- Apple

- Banana
- Orange
- Pineapple
- Orange squash
- Blueberry
- Greek yogurt
- Coffee powder
- 50 ml of fat free milk

Preparation method

1. Cut all fruits in to small pieces and put them into a bowl. Mix with Greek yogurt. Refrigerate for an hour.
2. Place the mixture of fruits and yogurt in the blender. Add milk, coffee powder, fruit mixture, orange squash and ice cubes as well. Blend them nicely till they form a smooth liquid.
3. Have it while chilled along with a vegetable sandwich to keep your fat content in check.

Tomato soup (post workout)

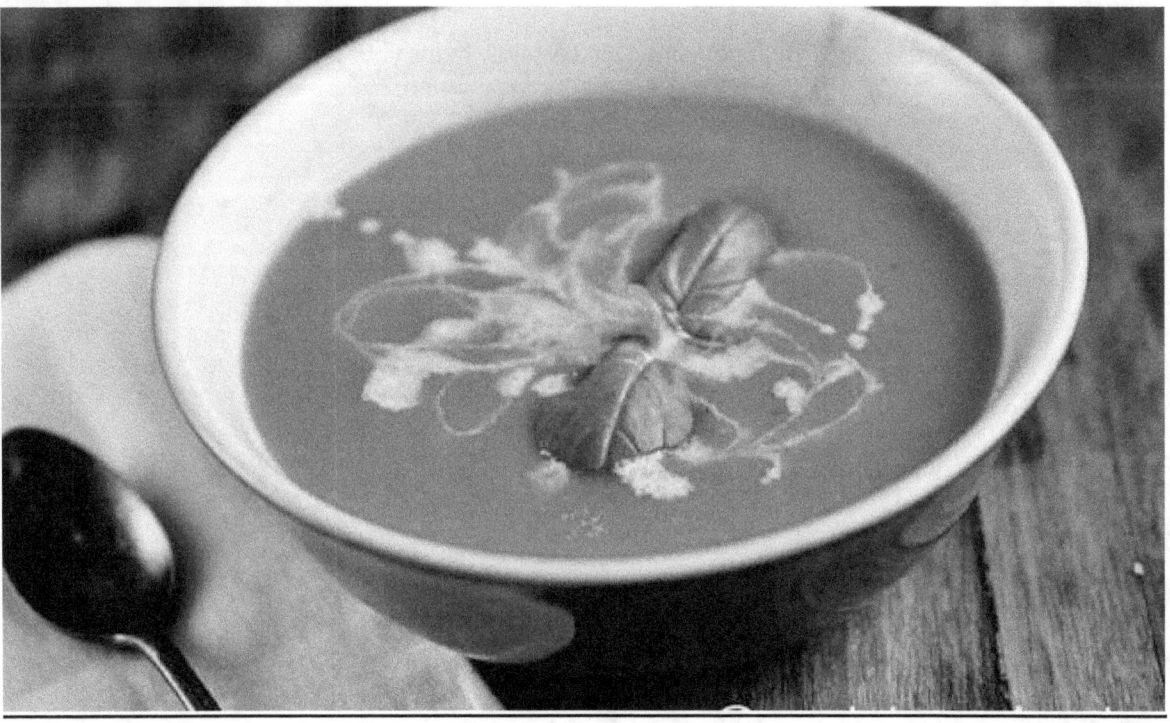

Ingredients

- A pound of tomatoes

- Broccoli
- Olive oil
- Salt
- Pepper
- Coriander
- Parsley
- 4 mint leaves
- Spring onions

Preparation method

1. Wash fresh tomatoes and make puree out of it.
2. Slice the broccoli, coriander, mint, parsley and spring onions into small pieces.
3. Put a cooking pot on flame and pour some of the olive oil.
4. Add tomato puree and all the diced vegetables.
5. You can also add any other leafy vegetables or other herbs you like.
6. Let the contents simmer on medium flame for 15 minutes.
7. Place the soup into a soup bowl. Add some bread crumbs and chopped coriander to garnish before serving.
8. Low calorie tomato soup is an appetizer which certainly helps your health.

Vegetable soup (post workout)

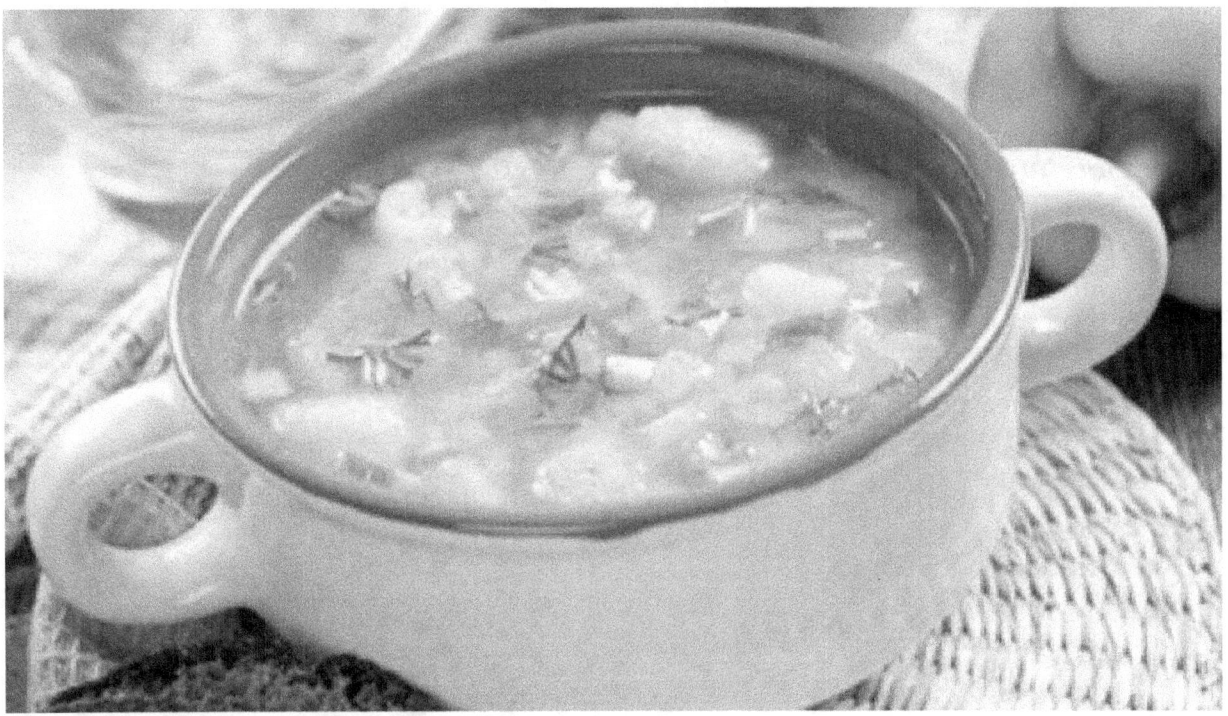

Ingredients

- Tomato
- Spinach
- Cabbage
- Broccoli
- Carrots
- salt pepper
- Onion
- Spring onions
- Zucchini
- Ginger garlic
- Chicken-broth

Preparation method

1. Finely chop all vegetables including spring onion, carrot, cabbage, one small tomato, ginger, garlic and spinach.
2. Place cooking pot on a medium flame and grease it lightly with extra virgin olive oil. Add onions, finely chopped ginger and garlic along with spring onions.
3. Stir it until the onions turn golden brown. Cumin seeds can be included if you like them.
4. Slowly pour the chicken broth and let it simmer for about 3 minutes on a high flame before you put in all the other vegetables.

5. Let it simmer on medium flame for 3 minutes now. Add salt and pepper to your taste and put out the flame.
6. Cook for 10 minutes before consuming.

Rice salad (post workout)

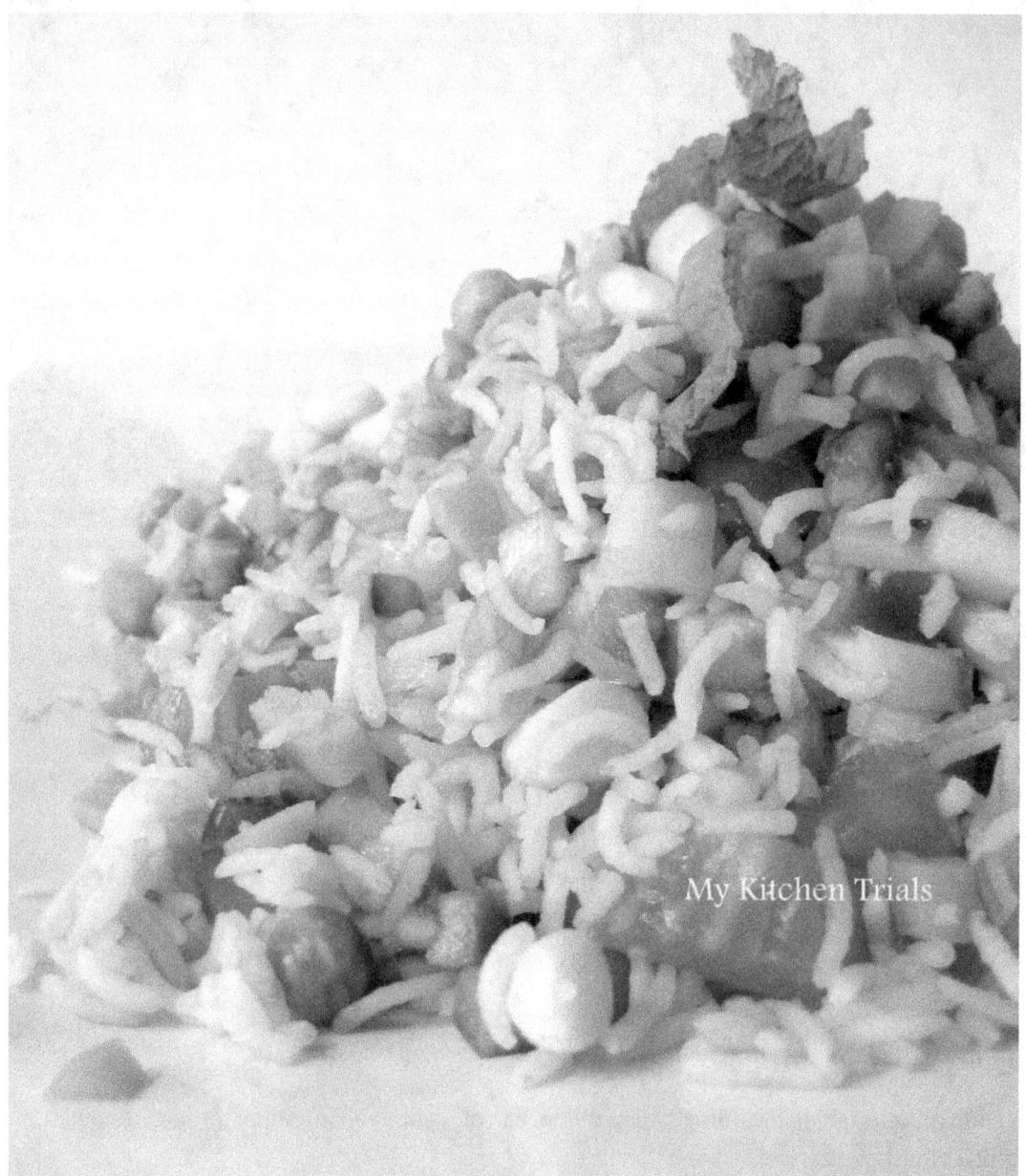

My Kitchen Trials

Ingredients

- Parsley
- Pepper
- Brown rice

- Salt
- corn
- Cumin seed turned into powder
- Spring onions
- Coriander
- Extra virgin olive oil
- Mint-leaves
- Carrot
- Chickpeas

<u>Preparation method</u>

1. Cook brown rice according to instructions, add turmeric to taste.
2. Keep the rice aside to cool so that the rice grains don't stick to each other.
3. Heat a cooking pan and grease it with olive oil. Put in finely chopped onions on medium flame until the onion turns to golden brown. Add 50 ml of vegetable broth, chick peas, carrots, parsley, corn, spring onions, salt and pepper.
4. Bring the seasoning to a low flame and mix it well into the cooled down brown rice. Add coriander for garnishing purpose before consuming.

These recipes can be varied slightly to suit your taste and cuisine but not to the extent where their core fat burning ingredients are altered.

Before you start burning fat

Fat burning process explained above is effective in general but as the saying goes "one size doesn't fit all". With respect to various parameters of the body such as sex, weight, height, body type and metabolism rate, the results vary. Crash diet is something which can lead to fatal conditions if not followed properly.

If the results are not satisfactory even after following the mentioned procedure accurately, please consult your nearest trainer who can advise after considering the above mentioned parameters of your body.

Quick fat reduction is just a myth. Consuming the mentioned food will not make you skinny without any exercise. Only a routine where a balance exercise such as cardio, zoomba, cycling, sprinting or strength training is combined with proper diet will give you results.

Starving the body to decrease the calorie intake will reduce your muscles. Rather slowly reduce the intake of calories while increasing calories spending so your body has a time to adapt. Also performing the same kind of exercise for a long time will not yield results as the body will adapt to these conditions. So exercises should be varied in types and also in intensity to give you maximum results.

The time period for training should not be too long as it leads to fatigue condition. Just do casual cardio until you get used to it and after that, intensity should be varied according to your discomfort level. Listen to your body. It will tell you when to stop and you should not perform until you are dead beat.

Start now; follow the routine exercise at least 4 to 5 times a week to maximize the results. Do not get discouraged if there are no satisfactory results at first, with patience and persistence you will get there eventually.

Burn the fat, live the dream.

Alicia Labert